CONNECT BIBLE STUDIES

The Lord of the Rings

J R R Tolkien
(HarperCollins)

Mission
Power
Wisdom and Guidance
Courage

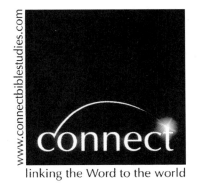

www.connectbiblestudies.com

connect

linking the Word to the world

CONNECT BIBLE STUDIES: The Lord of the Rings

Published in this format by Scripture Union, 207-209 Queensway, Bletchley, MK2 2EB, England.

Scripture Union is an international Christian charity working with churches in more than 130 countries providing resources to bring the good news about Jesus Christ to children, young people and families — and to encourage them to develop spiritually through the Bible and prayer.

As well as a network of volunteers, staff and associates who run holidays, church-based events and school Christian groups, Scripture Union produces a wide range of publications and supports those who use the resources through training programmes.

Email: info@scriptureunion.org.uk
Internet: www.scriptureunion.org.uk

© Damaris Trust, PO Box 200, Southampton, SO17 2DL.

Damaris Trust enables people to relate Christian faith and contemporary culture. It helps them to think about the issues within society from a Christian perspective and to explore God's truth as it is revealed in the Bible. Damaris provides resources via the Internet, workshops, publications and products.

Email: office@damaris.org
Internet: www.damaris.org

ALSO AVAILABLE AS AN ELECTRONIC DOWNLOAD: www.connectbiblestudies.com

Chief editor: Nick Pollard
Consultant Editor: Andrew Clark
Managing Editor: Di Archer
Written by Di Archer, James Murkett, Caroline Puntis, Tony Watkins

First published 2001; reprinted (twice) 2002
ISBN 1 85999 634 5

British Library Cataloguing-in-Publication Data: a catalogue record for this book is available from the British Library.

Cover design and print production by:
CPO, Garcia Estate, Canterbury Road, Worthing, West Sussex BN13 1BW.

Other titles in this series:

Harry Potter and the Goblet of Fire ISBN 1 85999 578 0
The Matrix ISBN 1 85999 579 9
U2: All that you can't leave behind ISBN 1 85999 580 2
Billy Elliot ISBN 1 85999 581 0
Chocolat ISBN 1 85999 608 6
Game Shows ISBN 1 85999 609 4
How to be Good ISBN 1 85999 610 8
Destiny's Child: Survivor ISBN 1 85999 613 2

AI (Artificial Intelligence) ISBN 1 85999 626 4
The Lord of the Rings ISBN 1 85999 634 5
The Simpsons ISBN 1 85999 529 2
Iris ISBN 1 85999 669 8
Dido: No Angel ISBN 1 85999 679 5
Sven-Göran Eriksson: On Football ISBN 1 85999 690 6
Superheroes ISBN 1 85999 702 3
The Pullman Trilogy: His Dark Materials ISBN 1 85999 714 7

And more titles following — check www.connectbiblestudies.com for latest titles or ask at any good Christian bookshop.

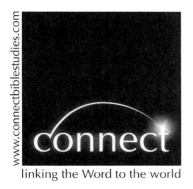

connect

linking the Word to the world

Using Connect Bible Studies

What Are These Studies?

These innovative home group Bible studies have two aims. Firstly, we design them to enable group members to dig into their Bibles and get to know them better. Secondly, we aim to help members to think through topical issues in a Biblical way. Hence the studies are based on a current popular book or film etc. The issues raised by these are the subjects for the Bible studies.

We do not envisage that all members will always be able to watch the films or read the books, or indeed that they will always want to. A summary is always provided. However, our vision is that knowing about these films and books empowers Christians to engage with friends and colleagues about them. Addressing issues from a Biblical perspective gives Christians confidence that they know what they think, and can bring a distinctive angle to bear in conversations.

The studies are produced in sets of four — i.e. four weeks' worth of group Bible Study material. These are available in print published by Scripture Union from your local Christian bookshop, or via the Internet at www.connectbiblestudies.com. Anyone can sign up for a free monthly email newsletter that announces the new studies and provides other information (sign up on the Connect Bible Studies website at www.connectbiblestudies.com/uk/register).

How Do I Use Them?

We design the studies to stimulate creative thought and discussion within a Biblical context. Each section therefore has a range of questions or options from which you as leader may choose in order to tailor the study to your group's needs and desires. Different approaches may appeal at different times, so the studies aim to supply lots of choice. Whilst adhering to the main aim of corporate Bible study, some types of questions may enable this for your group better than others — so take your pick.

Group members should be supplied with the appropriate sheet that they can fill in, each one also showing the relevant summary.

Leader's notes contain:

1. Opening Questions

These help your group settle in to discussion, whilst introducing the topics. They may be straightforward, personal or creative, but are aiming to provoke a response.

2. Summary

We suggest the summary of the book or film will follow now, read aloud if necessary. There may well be reactions that group members want to express even before getting on to the week's issue.

3. Key Issue

Again, either read from the leader's notes, or summarised.

4. Bible Study

Lots of choice here. Choose as appropriate to suit your group — get digging into the Bible. Background reading and texts for further help and study are suggested, but please use the material provided to inspire your group to explore their Bibles as much as possible. A concordance might be a handy standby for looking things up. A commentary could be useful too, such as the *New Bible Commentary 21st Century Edition* (IVP, 1994). The idea is to help people to engage with the truth of God's word, wrestling with it if necessary but making it their own.

Don't plan to work through every question here. Within each section the two questions explore roughly the same ground but from different angles or in different ways. Our advice is to take one question from each section. The questions are open-ended so each ought to yield good discussion — though of course any discussion in a Bible study may need prompting to go a little further.

5. Implications

Here the aim is to tie together the perspectives gained through Bible study and the impact of the book or film. The implications may be personal, a change in worldview, or new ideas for relating to non-churchgoers. Choose questions that adapt to the flow of the discussion.

6. Prayer

Leave time for it! We suggest a time of open prayer, or praying in pairs if the group would prefer. Encourage your members to focus on issues from your study that had a particular impact on them. Try different approaches to prayer — light a candle, say a prayer each, write prayers down, play quiet worship music — aim to facilitate everyone to relate to God.

7. Background Reading

You will find links to some background reading on the Connect Bible Studies website: www.connectbiblestudies.com/

8. Online Discussion

You can discuss the studies online with others on the Connect Bible Studies website at www.connectbiblestudies.com/discuss/

Scriptures referred to are taken from the Holy Bible, New International Version (NIV). Copyright © 1973, 1978, 1984 by International Bible Society. Other Bible translations can, of course, be used for the studies and having a range of translations in a group can be helpful and useful in discussion.

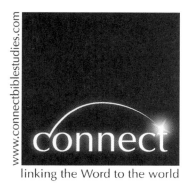

The Lord of the Rings

By J R R Tolkien (HarperCollins)

Part One: Mission

'I am not made for perilous quests. I wish I had never seen the Ring!
Why did it come to me? Why was I chosen?'
Frodo (Book I, The Shadow of the Past)

Please read Using Connect Bible Studies *before leading a Bible study using this material.*

Opening Questions

Choose one of these questions.

Have you ever dreaded a task that you know you must do?	What do you think was the hardest part of Frodo's mission?
Do you tackle difficult jobs first or put them off? Why?	What is the hardest thing someone has ever asked you to do?

Summary

Frodo Baggins lives in the pleasant surroundings of the Shire, in the northwestern lands of Middle-earth. Like all hobbits, he enjoys the comfort of good food and a well-earned smoke. Following the sudden departure of his cousin Bilbo, Frodo inherits many riches — including a mysterious gold ring.

The wise wizard Gandalf explains the story of the ring to its new owner: long ago, Sauron the Great made it on the Fire-mountain, Orodruin. He was overthrown by the last great alliance of elves and men, one of whom subsequently lost the ring. Gandalf reveals to Frodo that this is the One Ring that could completely restore the power of the Dark Lord and give him command over all lesser rings. An inscription bears the key to its power: 'One Ring to rule them all, One Ring to find them / One Ring to bring them all and in the darkness bind them.' This Ring must be returned to the only fire great enough to destroy it — as Ring-bearer, Frodo is called to deliver it into the Cracks of Doom on Orodruin, far away in Sauron's dark lands in the South.

Nothing could be less desirable to Frodo than leaving the safety and comfort of the Shire. Gandalf says that he is ready to support him, if he chooses to go: 'The decision lies with you. But I will always help you ... I will help you bear this burden, as long as it is yours to bear.' Frodo accepts the call and sets out.

Key Issue: Mission

Frodo is less than delighted to discover that he is the one who must deal with the Ring. Like many of us, he does not thrill to the task he must perform. It involves danger and sacrifice, with no guarantee of success. Having responded to the call to serve God, Christians are commissioned to obey his specific challenges to us. What does the Bible say about our readiness to follow God no matter what? And where does duty come in? How can we be encouraged to persevere? Who or what can inspire us to keep going?

Bible Study

Choose one question from each section. You may like to follow the questions centred on Jesus.

1. Calling

> *'I too once passed the Dimril Gate,' said Aragorn quietly; 'but though I also came out again, the memory is very evil. I do not wish to enter Moria a second time.'*
> *'And I don't wish to enter it even once,' said Pippin.*
> *'Nor me,' muttered Sam.*
> *'Of course not!' said Gandalf. 'Who would? But the question is: who will follow me, if I lead you there?'*
> *'I will,' said Gimli eagerly.*
> *'I will,' said Aragorn heavily.* (Book II, A Journey in the Dark)

♦ Read Exodus 3:4–15 and 4:1–17. Why did Moses question God's call? How did God answer him?

♦ Read Luke 4:14–30. What was Jesus' mission? What difficulties did he encounter?

Leaders: The widow and Naaman were not Israelites — redemption is not just for the Jews, which is what Jesus' hearers would have been expecting.

4:14-21 = Jesus' mission
22 - 30 = difficulties - ppl in his home-town did not hear what he was saying

His message was repulsive to them - redemption for all!

2. Duty — prepared to suffer

'But I count you blessed, Gimli son of Glóin: for your loss you suffer of your own free will, and you might have chosen otherwise. But you have not forsaken your companions, and the least reward that you shall have is that the memory of Lothlórien shall remain ever clear and unstained in your heart, and shall neither fade nor grow stale.' (Legolas, Book II, Farewell to Lórien)

♦ Read Jeremiah 38:1–28. How did Jeremiah fulfil his duty to God? What were the consequences?

Leaders: You may like to consider how this commission would have been hard for Jeremiah.

♦ Mark 8:27–38. What was Jesus' attitude to the suffering ahead of him? What are the implications for those who follow him?

v 32 - he spoke plainly - accepting
v 34 - take up cross - himself - saves his life will lose it - burden - denial of self

3. Readiness

'But so far my only thought has been to get here; and I hope I shan't have to go any further. It is very pleasant just to rest. I have had a month of exile and adventure, and I find that has been as much as I want.' (Frodo, Book II, Many Meetings)

♦ Read Acts 8:26–40. How is Philip's attitude of readiness apparent throughout the passage? In what different ways was God at work?

he had compassion - sheep without a shepherd.

helps her woman

♦ Read Mark 1:35–39; 5:21–34; 6:30–34 and John 4:4–10. What does Jesus make of these interruptions? Who and what was he responding to?

)- he went to the villages preach - responding to everyone'

Leaders: You may find it helpful to refer back to Jesus' calling in Luke 4:18, 19.

Responding to need

4. Perseverance

Sam drew a deep breath. There was a path, but how he was to get up the slope to it he did not know ... Suddenly a sense of urgency which he did not understand came to Sam. It was almost as if he had been called: 'Now, now, or it will be too late!' He braced himself and got up. (Book VI, Mount Doom)

♦ Read 2 Timothy 4:1–22. How and why does Paul encourage us to persevere?

♦ Read Luke 22:39–46. What was the essence of Jesus' dilemma? How did his choice demonstrate perseverance?

he sweated blood. strengthened by a angel prayed so that he would't fall in2 temptation

↘ he didn't want 2 do what God had asked him 2
↘ not my will but yours.

Implications

'So that was the job I felt I had to do when I started,' thought Sam: 'to help Mr Frodo to the last step and then die with him? Well, if that is the job then I must do it.'
(Book VI, Mount Doom)

Choose one or more of the following questions.

♦ How can we encourage each other to be obedient to God when we don't feel like it?

♦ Is God calling you to do something challenging? Are you ready for the cost?

♦ How do we know what God is calling us to do?

♦ Is duty still a valid concept in our please-yourself culture?

♦ What helps you to persevere when the going gets tough?

♦ Have you given up on something you wish you hadn't? Can you make a new start with God's help?

♦ How can the idea of calling help us to encourage those who lack direction in life?

Prayer

Spend some time praying through these issues.

Background Reading

You will find links to some background reading on the Connect Bible Studies website: www.connectbiblestudies.com/uk/catalogue/0010/background.htm

Discuss

Discuss this study in the online discussion forums at www.connectbiblestudies.com/discuss

Members' Sheet: Mission — Part 1

Summary

Frodo Baggins lives in the pleasant surroundings of the Shire, in the northwestern lands of Middle-earth. Like all hobbits, he enjoys the comfort of good food and a well-earned smoke. Following the sudden departure of his cousin Bilbo, Frodo inherits many riches — including a mysterious gold ring.

The wise wizard Gandalf explains the story of the ring to its new owner: long ago, Sauron the Great made it on the Fire-mountain, Orodruin. He was overthrown by the last great alliance of elves and men, one of whom subsequently lost the ring. Gandalf reveals to Frodo that this is the One Ring that could completely restore the power of the Dark Lord and give him command over all lesser rings. An inscription bears the key to its power: 'One Ring to rule them all, One Ring to find them / One Ring to bring them all and in the darkness bind them.' This Ring must be returned to the only fire great enough to destroy it — as Ring-bearer, Frodo is called to deliver it into the Cracks of Doom on Orodruin, far away in Sauron's dark lands in the South.

Nothing could be less desirable to Frodo than leaving the safety and comfort of the Shire. Gandalf says that he is ready to support him, if he chooses to go: 'The decision lies with you. But I will always help you ... I will help you bear this burden, as long as it is yours to bear.' Frodo accepts the call and sets out.

Key Issue

Bible Study notes

Implications

Prayer

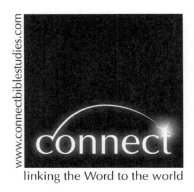

www.connectbiblestudies.com

connect
linking the Word to the world

The Lord of the Rings

By J R R Tolkien (HarperCollins)

Part Two: Power

The two powers strove in him. For a moment, perfectly balanced between their piercing points, he writhed, tormented. Suddenly he was aware of himself again. Frodo, neither the Voice nor the Eye: free to choose and with one remaining instant in which to do so.
(Book II, The Breaking of the Fellowship)

Please read Using Connect Bible Studies *before leading a Bible study using this material.*

Opening Questions

Choose one of these questions.

'Power corrupts and absolute power corrupts absolutely.' Do you agree?	Who do you think is the most powerful person in the country and why?
Who is the most powerful character in *The Lord of the Rings*?	Is having power a good thing or a bad thing? Why?

Summary

Frodo the hobbit's mission is to see that a powerful ring does not get into the hands of Sauron the Great, the Dark Lord. On his finger, the Ring would give him power so terrible that no good would be able to resist it. The Ring must be destroyed in the fires of Mount Doom, on Sauron's doorstep in Mordor where his power is strongest.

The power of the Ring itself works evil amongst the Company sent with Frodo to complete the mission. Boromir has been influenced by the will of the Dark Lord and is now persuaded that in his hands the Ring would only be used for good. Seeing the potential for corruption, Frodo breaks the Fellowship and continues with only Sam for support. They are trailed by the troublesome Gollum, once the Ring-bearer himself and still captive to its power. Once in Mordor, Frodo's will is gradually smothered. As he stands over the Cracks of Doom, Frodo cannot destroy the Ring. Gollum attacks him and manages to bite off Frodo's finger with the Ring still intact. He stumbles and falls into the fires. Sauron's power is destroyed.

The King returns to his throne and uses his power to restore the country. The hobbits finally go home to their beloved Shire, only to find that Saruman, once a great and wise wizard who turned to evil, has infiltrated and taken over. However, without Sauron he is nothing — as Frodo banishes him from the Shire, his own servant kills him.

Key Issue: Power

In *The Lord of the Rings*, Gandalf is afraid of touching the infamous Ring in case its power should prove too much and corrupt him. His companions must destroy the Ring before the Dark Lord can get hold of it. The Ring is power. It is so powerful that it can even corrupt the good. So our study focuses on what the Bible says about power. Does it acknowledge that power can be used wrongly? What does it teach about the right use of power? And if there is a right and a wrong use, how do we know exactly which side we are on?

Bible Study

Choose one question from each section. You may like to follow the questions centred on Jesus.

1.   Good use

In the days that followed his crowning the King sat on his throne in the Hall of the Kings and pronounced judgements ... and all was healed and made good ...
(Book VI, The Steward and the King)

♦   Read 2 Kings 23:1–11, 21–25. How did Josiah use his power for good? What was he trying to achieve and why?

Leaders: Unlike many of the previous Kings of Judah, Josiah sought to follow God. During his reign, the Book of the Law was rediscovered during repairs on the Temple at Jerusalem. Upon reading the Book, Josiah was moved by the disobedience of Judah and was concerned about God's coming judgement against such sin (2 Kings 22).

♦   Read John 5:1–30. What is the nature of Jesus' power? What does and does not limit his use of power?

2. Bad use

'But it's these Men, Sam, the Chief's Men. He sends them round everywhere, and if any of us small folk stand up for our rights, they drag him off to the Lockholes.'
(Robin Smallburrow, Book VI, The Scouring of the Shire)

♦ Read Ezekiel 11:1–15. How were the people of Jerusalem exploiting their position? Why did they think they could?

Leaders: Ezekiel is speaking against the leaders left behind in Jerusalem (the cooking pot) after the Babylonians took many into exile. It appears that they thought they were 'the meat', meaning the choice portions kept safe in the pot, while those in exile were discarded and worthless. Ezekiel reinterprets 'the meat' to refer to the innocents killed by these leaders. No longer will the city be a cooking pot keeping the leaders safe — they are now under God's judgment and are about to be picked out of the pot and discarded.

♦ Read Luke 11:37–54. How were the Pharisees and experts in the law abusing their power? How had this abuse affected them and others?

3. Restraint

Sam's hand wavered. His mind was hot with wrath and the memory of evil. It would be just to slay this treacherous, murderous creature, just and many times deserved; and also it seemed the only safe thing to do. But deep in his heart there was something that restrained him: he could not strike this thing lying in the dust, forlorn, ruinous, utterly wretched. (Book VI, Mount Doom)

♦ Read Genesis 50:15–21. What opportunity did Joseph have to avenge the past? Why did he show restraint?

Leaders: Joseph had been sold into slavery by his brothers many years before. Joseph had previously assured them that he saw God's hand at work in his situation and had urged them not to be distressed (Gen 45:4–13). However, it seems that the brothers were unsure as to Joseph's feelings towards them.

♦ Read Mark 10:35–45. What was wrong with James' and John's question? What does Jesus teach and show about power and authority?

4. Whose side are you on anyway?

'Do not kill him even now. For [Saruman] has not hurt me. And in any case I do not wish him to be slain in this evil mood. He was great once, of a noble kind that we should not dare to raise our hands against. He is fallen, and his cure is beyond us; but I would still spare him, in the hope that he may find it.' (Frodo, Book VI, The Scouring of the Shire)

- Read Ezekiel 33:10–20. What are the warnings and encouragements in this passage? How will all power struggles ultimately be resolved?

- Read Mark 3:1–35. How do the different groups respond to Jesus? What is the issue at stake?

Implications

'Other evils there are that may come; for Sauron is himself but a servant or emissary. Yet it is not our part to master all the tides of the world, but to do what is in us for the succour of those years wherein we are set, uprooting the evil in the fields that we know, so that those who live after may have clean earth to till. What weather they shall have is not ours to rule.' (Gandalf, Book V, The Last Debate)

Choose one or more of the following questions.

- Are you in a position of power over others, e.g. at work or in the home? How can you use your position to bless and do good to them?

- Most of us are victims of abuse of power by others in some way or another — are there issues you need to deal with, people you need to forgive?

- Rather than 'lording it over' one another, how can we encourage each other to find our significance in God?

- Why is power so attractive? How can we guard against wanting it for wrong reasons?

- We may have been Christians for years or a day, but there are some choices that we still have to make daily. In what areas of your life do you have a power struggle?

- In what ways does Jesus use power perfectly, and how can we follow his example?

Prayer

Spend some time praying through these issues.

Background Reading

You will find links to some background reading on the Connect Bible Studies website: www.connectbiblestudies.com/uk/catalogue/0010/background.htm

Discuss

Discuss this study in the online discussion forums at www.connectbiblestudies.com/discuss

Members' Sheet: Power — Part 2

Summary

Frodo the hobbit's mission is to see that a powerful ring does not get into the hands of Sauron the Great, the Dark Lord. On his finger, the Ring would give him power so terrible that no good would be able to resist it. The Ring must be destroyed in the fires of Mount Doom, on Sauron's doorstep in Mordor where his power is strongest.

The power of the Ring itself works evil amongst the Company sent with Frodo to complete the mission. Boromir has been influenced by the will of the Dark Lord and is now persuaded that in his hands the Ring would only be used for good. Seeing the potential for corruption, Frodo breaks the Fellowship and continues with only Sam for support. They are trailed by the troublesome Gollum, once the Ring-bearer himself and still captive to its power. Once in Mordor, Frodo's will is gradually smothered. As he stands over the Cracks of Doom, Frodo cannot destroy the Ring. Gollum attacks him and manages to bite off Frodo's finger with the Ring still intact. He stumbles and falls into the fires. Sauron's power is destroyed.

The King returns to his throne and uses his power to restore the country. The hobbits finally go home to their beloved Shire, only to find that Saruman, once a great and wise wizard who turned to evil, has infiltrated and taken over. However, without Sauron he is nothing — as Frodo banishes him from the Shire, his own servant kills him.

Key Issue

Bible Study notes

Implications

Prayer

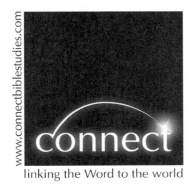

www.connectbiblestudies.com

connect
linking the Word to the world

The Lord of the Rings

By J R R Tolkien (HarperCollins)

Part Three: Wisdom and Guidance

'Let the guide go first while you have one.'
Aragorn (Book II, A Journey in the Dark)

Please read Using Connect Bible Studies *before leading a Bible study using this material.*

Opening Questions

Choose one of these questions.

Who is the wisest person you know, and what makes them so?	What is wisdom?
Who do you go to for advice and why?	Who do you consider to be the wisest person in *The Lord of the Rings*?

Summary

Frodo needs all the help he can get for his dangerous mission to the fires of Mount Doom. He bears a powerful ring which must be destroyed in order to defeat Sauron, the Dark Lord. Gandalf the wizard is at hand with much wise counsel, for he understands the power of the Ring and the many different peoples and paths that Frodo will encounter on his way. He commissions Aragorn to lead Frodo to Rivendell, where he must first appear before the Council of Elrond the elf-lord. The Council decides that a Fellowship should accompany Frodo and do all within their power to see that the mission is completed.

When they come to a long mountain range, Aragorn and Gandalf disagree on the path they should follow. Fear gets the better of the majority and the Company ventures up a high mountain pass, only to be stopped by the ravages of storm and snow. They retrace their steps and follow Gandalf into the bowels of the dreaded Moria. In a ferocious battle with some of Sauron's servants, Gandalf is lost. Aragorn takes over as guide, but all the Company misses Gandalf's profound and fearless wisdom.

When Gandalf returns he finds the Fellowship broken — Frodo and Sam struggle on with the Ring whilst the rest of the Company prepare for war. Gandalf then leads the armies of the West into the very hands of the enemy, yet still his wisdom prevails — the Dark Lord's eye is turned away as Frodo completes his mission.

Key Issue: Wisdom

As Frodo and friends start out on their perilous adventure, they are desperate for someone to guide them who knows more than they do about the challenges that lie ahead. Knowing which way to turn and what to do when things get difficult becomes a matter of life and death. They need wisdom. Knowledge is all very well, but, as the hobbits discover, it is applying it in the right way that counts. There are probably many people who would admit that the Bible is a source of wisdom, but how many actually use it? In this study, we look at what wisdom is, where we get it from, and what difference it can make to our lives.

Bible Study

Choose one question from each section. You may like to follow the questions centred on Jesus.

1. Why wisdom?

'I've made up my mind,' [Sam] kept saying to himself. But he had not. Though he had done his best to think it out, what he was doing was altogether against the grain of his nature. 'Have I got it wrong?' he muttered. 'What ought I to have done?'
(Book IV, The Choices of Master Samwise)

- ◆ Read Proverbs 8:1–36. What is wisdom? How is it essential to life?

- ◆ Read Matthew 11:25–30. Why is it wise to come to Jesus? How is his burden light?

2. Sources of wisdom — people

'Elves seldom give unguarded advice, for advice is a dangerous gift, even from the wise to the wise, and all courses may run ill. But what would you? You have not told me all concerning yourself; and how then shall I choose better than you? But if you demand advice, I will for friendship's sake give it.' (Gildor, Book I, Three is Company)

- ◆ Psalm 1:1–6. What choices do we have in obtaining guidance? Contrast the ways of the righteous and the wicked, and where they end.

♦ Read Luke 6:37–45. To whom does Jesus say we should - and should not - go for advice? How do we become wise counsellors?

3. Sources of wisdom — God

'Do not be afraid! I have been with him on many a journey, if never on one so dark; and there are tales of Rivendell of greater deeds of his than any that I have seen. He will not go astray — if there is any path to find. He has led us here against our fears, but he will lead us out again, at whatever cost to himself.'
(Aragorn on Gandalf, Book II, A Journey in the Dark)

♦ Read Job 28:1–28. What is true wisdom? What value does it have?

♦ Read Isaiah 11:1–5. What is Spirit-given wisdom? What does this messianic figure take into account when he judges?

Leaders: This is a Messianic prophecy explaining that Jesus will come from David's line. He will act and judge with true righteousness and insight.

4. Wisdom in action

'Come, Aragorn son of Arathorn!' [Gandalf] said. 'Do not regret your choice in the valley of the Emyn Muil, nor call it a vain pursuit. You chose amid doubts the path that seemed right: the choice was just, and it has been rewarded. For so we have met in time, who otherwise might have met too late.' (Book III, The White Rider)

♦ Read Isaiah 30:15–22. What was God's reaction to Israel's past mistakes? What is the way of wisdom for the future?

♦ Read Luke 6:46–49. What is the fundamental difference between these builders? What point was Jesus making about the guidance he gives?

Implications

'Well, Frodo,' said Aragorn at last. 'I fear that the burden is laid upon you. You are the Bearer appointed by the Council. Your own way you alone can choose. In this matter I cannot advise you. I am not Gandalf, and though I have tried to bear his part, I do not know what design or hope he had for this hour, if indeed he had any. Most likely it seems that if he were here now the choice would still wait on you. Such is your fate.'
(Book II, The Breaking of the Fellowship)

Choose one or more of the following questions.

- ◆ Are there any choices we make that do not really matter?

- ◆ How do you know when God is guiding you?

- ◆ Do you tend to ask people for advice whom you know will agree with your opinion?

- ◆ How do we grow in wisdom?

- ◆ What is the wisest way to make big decisions?

- ◆ What would you say to a friend who relies on horoscopes and magazines, etc., to make decisions?

Prayer

Spend some time praying through these issues.

Background Reading

You will find links to some background reading on the Connect Bible Studies website: www.connectbiblestudies.com/uk/catalogue/0010/background.htm

Discuss

Discuss this study in the online discussion forums at www.connectbiblestudies.com/discuss

Members' Sheet: Wisdom and Guidance — Part 3

Summary

Frodo needs all the help he can get for his dangerous mission to the fires of Mount Doom. He bears a powerful ring which must be destroyed in order to defeat Sauron, the Dark Lord. Gandalf the wizard is at hand with much wise counsel, for he understands the power of the Ring and the many different peoples and paths that Frodo will encounter on his way. He commissions Aragorn to lead Frodo to Rivendell, where he must first appear before the Council of Elrond the elf-lord. The Council decides that a Fellowship should accompany Frodo and do all within their power to see that the mission is completed.

When they come to a long mountain range, Aragorn and Gandalf disagree on the path they should follow. Fear gets the better of the majority and the Company ventures up a high mountain pass, only to be stopped by the ravages of storm and snow. They retrace their steps and follow Gandalf into the bowels of the dreaded Moria. In a ferocious battle with some of Sauron's servants, Gandalf is lost. Aragorn takes over as guide, but all the Company misses Gandalf's profound and fearless wisdom.

When Gandalf returns he finds the Fellowship broken — Frodo and Sam struggle on with the Ring whilst the rest of the Company prepare for war. Gandalf then leads the armies of the West into the very hands of the enemy, yet still his wisdom prevails — the Dark Lord's eye is turned away as Frodo completes his mission.

Key Issue

Bible Study notes

Implications

Prayer

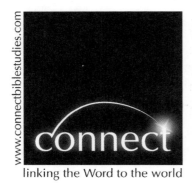

www.connectbiblestudies.com

connect
linking the Word to the world

The Lord of the Rings

By J R R Tolkien (HarperCollins)

Part Four: Courage

There is a seed of courage hidden (often deeply, it is true) in the heart of the fattest and most timid hobbit, waiting for some final and desperate danger to make it grow. Frodo was neither very fat nor very timid; indeed, though he did not know it, Bilbo (and Gandalf) had thought him the best hobbit in the Shire.
(Book I, Fog on the Barrow-downs)

Please read Using Connect Bible Studies *before leading a Bible study using this material.*

Opening Questions

Choose one of these questions.

What is the bravest thing you have ever done?	Have you ever regretted not rising to a challenge?
Who do you think is the most courageous character in *The Lord of the Rings*?	'Courage is feeling afraid and going on anyway.' Do you agree? Why?

Summary

Having agreed to take on the mission to return the dangerous Ring to its birthplace for destruction, Frodo wonders how he will manage the task alone. He is relieved when three of his friends set out with him, and encouraged later by the forming of a Fellowship who will share his burden of responsibility.

The Ring has enough power to corrupt even the strongest will. When Frodo detects the danger it presents to the rest of the Fellowship, he decides to continue alone. Sam cannot bear the thought of his master being on his own and tries to guess which way he will go. He catches up with him in the nick of time and the pair set off together. As they enter Mordor, where the evil power is strongest, the Ring becomes heavy around Frodo's neck. Faithful Sam would carry the Ring himself, but this is the one way that he cannot serve his master.

The going is tough and several times Sam forgoes his portion of rationed food for love of his master. Although Frodo's will has got them this far, the power of Mordor slowly saps his strength away. Sam picks him up and carries him. When finally the mission is complete, Frodo and Sam are whisked away to safety. After they have rested they find that they are indeed the heroes of the War against the Lord of the Rings — and that their courage saved the day.

Key Issue: Courage

There was no doubt in Frodo's mind that his mission to deal with the Ring was unwelcome. He would much rather have stayed at home in the Shire and known nothing about it. Yet, when it came to the crunch he took his responsibility seriously and set off into the unknown with the Ring. Frodo is not alone in facing situations which call for courage. None of us seem to escape times of challenge. Are we called to be brave on our own, or can the Bible help us? Does God acknowledge our need for encouragement? Who in the Bible can inspire us when we are up against it? Does being courageous really make a difference to anything?

Bible Study

Choose one question from each section. You may like to follow the questions centred on Jesus.

1. In need of courage

> *The Nazgûl came again, and as their Dark Lord now grew and put forth his strength, so their voices, which uttered only his will and his malice, were filled with evil and horror. At length even the stout-hearted would fling themselves to the ground as the hidden menace passed over them, or they would stand, letting their weapons fall from nerveless hands while into their minds a blackness came, and they thought no more of war, but only on hiding and of crawling, and of death.* (Book V, The Siege of Gondor)

♦   Read Numbers 13:17–14:4. Which interpretation of the spies' report was easier to believe? What conclusions did the people jump to?

Leaders: Moses had commanded a party of spies to go and survey the land of Canaan. God had promised them the land, but the people had other ideas.

♦   Read Matthew 8:23–27. Why were the disciples afraid? How did Jesus change everything?

Leaders: Some of the disciples were experienced fishermen and had doubtless sailed on the same lake in storm conditions. Yet something about this storm and its intensity led them to think that their lives were in danger.

2. Being Encouraged

'I will tread the path with you, Gandalf!' said Gimli. 'I will go and look on the halls of Durin, whatever may wait there — if you can find the doors that are shut.'
'Good, Gimli!' said Gandalf. 'You encourage me. We will seek the hidden doors together. And we will come through.' (Book II, A Journey in the Dark)

- ◆ Read Joshua 1:1–18. What is the nature of the encouragement Joshua received? How was it designed to help?

- ◆ Read Mark 1:9–13. How did God encourage Jesus? How was the timing of this encouragement significant?

3. Courage in action

Frodo rose to his feet. A great weariness was on him, but his will was firm and his heart lighter. He spoke aloud to himself. 'I will do now what I must,' he said. 'This at least is plain: the evil of the Ring is already at work even in the Company, and the Ring must leave them before it does more harm. I will go alone ... At once.'
(Book II, The Breaking of the Fellowship)

- ◆ Read Judges 7:1–25. How does God compel Gideon to trust him? What are the results?

   Leaders: God had called Gideon to defeat Midian. He decided to assemble an army but God had a different plan. Those soldiers who remained standing at the river and lapped showed that they were prepared for an emergency.

- ◆ Read Luke 9:51 and Matthew 27:1–14. Compare the perspectives and actions of Jesus and Judas.

4. Heroes

And then to Sam's surprise and utter confusion [Aragorn] bowed his knee before them; and taking them by the hand, Frodo upon his right and Sam upon his left, he led them to the throne, and setting them upon it, he turned to the men and captains who stood by and spoke, so that his voice rang over all the host, crying:
'Praise them with great praise!' (Book VI, The Field of Cormallen)

- ◆ Read Joshua 23:1–16. What does Joshua's speech tell us about the kind of man he was? What does he remind the Israelites about?

- ◆ Read Hebrews 12:1–3. How is Jesus the ultimate hero?

Implications

'The brave things in the old tales and songs, Mr Frodo: adventures, as I used to call them. I used to think that they were things the wonderful folk of the stories went out and looked for, because they wanted them, because they were exciting and life was a bit dull, a kind of sport, as you might say. But that's not the way of it with the tales that really mattered, or the ones that stay in the mind. Folk seem to have been just landed in them, usually — their paths were laid that way, as you put it. But I expect they had lots of chances, like us, of turning back, only they didn't. And if they had, we shouldn't know, because they'd have been forgotten...' (Sam, Book IV, The Stairs of Cirith Ungol)

Choose one or more of the following questions.

- Even Jesus needed encouragement. How can we encourage each other more?

- Why do things often seem to get difficult when we are going God's way?
  Refiners fire.

- How would you talk to a friend about their heroes in *The Lord of the Rings*, and your real heroes?

- Does courage make a difference? Does it matter if we back out of challenges?

- What qualities do you value in your heroes, and how can you be more like them?

- If you are facing seemingly impossible challenges just now, how can your group encourage and help you?

Prayer

Spend some time praying through these issues.

Background Reading

You will find links to some background reading on the Connect Bible Studies website: www.connectbiblestudies.com/uk/catalogue/0010/background.htm

Discuss

Discuss this study in the online discussion forums at www.connectbiblestudies.com/discuss

Members' Sheet: Courage — Part 4

Summary

Having agreed to take on the mission to return the dangerous Ring to its birthplace for destruction, Frodo wonders how he will manage the task alone. He is relieved when three of his friends set out with him, and encouraged later by the forming of a Fellowship who will share his burden of responsibility.

The Ring has enough power to corrupt even the strongest will. When Frodo detects the danger it presents to the rest of the Fellowship, he decides to continue alone. Sam cannot bear the thought of his master being on his own and tries to guess which way he will go. He catches up with him in the nick of time and the pair set off together. As they enter Mordor, where the evil power is strongest, the Ring becomes heavy around Frodo's neck. Faithful Sam would carry the Ring himself, but this is the one way that he cannot serve his master.

The going is tough and several times Sam forgoes his portion of rationed food for love of his master. Although Frodo's will has got them this far, the power of Mordor slowly saps his strength away. Sam picks him up and carries him. When finally the mission is complete, Frodo and Sam are whisked away to safety. After they have rested they find that they are indeed the heroes of the War against the Lord of the Rings — and that their courage saved the day.

Key Issue

Bible Study notes

Implications

Prayer